Sudden, Unexplained Infant Death Investigation

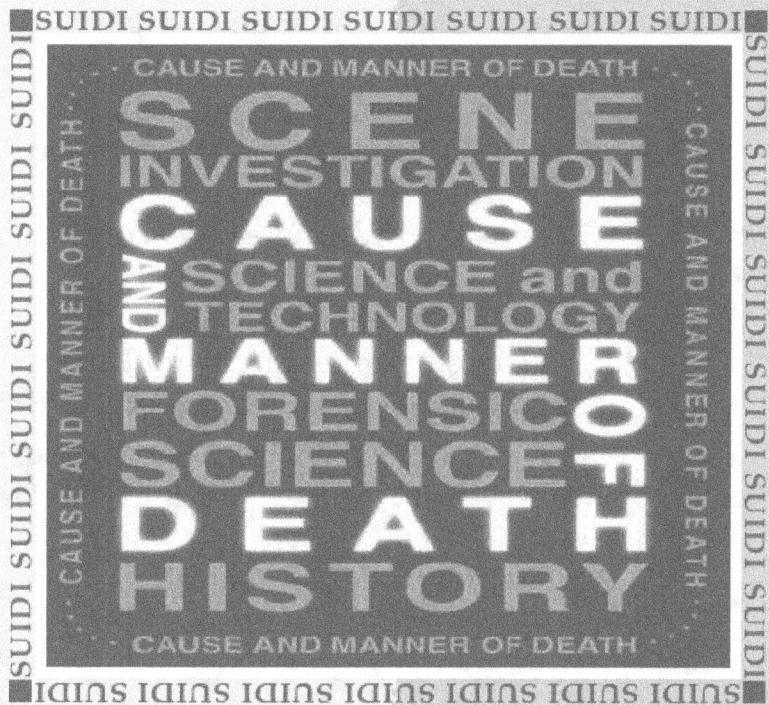

Infant Death Investigation:
Guidelines for the Scene Investigator

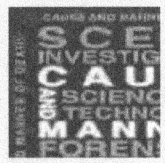

DEPARTMENT OF HEALTH AND HUMAN SERVICES
Maternal and Infant Health Branch
Division of Reproductive Health
Centers for Disease Control and Prevention
Atlanta, Georgia 30333

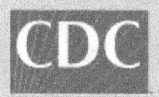

Project Funding Provided by the
Centers for Disease Control and Prevention
Atlanta, Georgia
Contract #200-2005-13514

Randy L. Hanzlick, MD
Chief Medical Examiner
Fulton County Medical Examiners Office
Atlanta, Georgia

Jeffrey M. Jentzen, MD
Chief Medical Examiner
Milwaukee County Medical Examiners Office
Milwaukee, Wisconsin

Steven C. Clark, PhD
Director of Research and Development
National Association of Medical Examiners
Educational Consultant
American Board of Medicolegal Death Investigators

This information handbook is intended as a guide to recommended practices the investigating infant deaths and reporting scene data to the pathologist. It is not intended to take the place of existing laws or regulations.

Sudden, Unexplained InfantDeathInvestigation

Guidelines for the Scene Investigator

Approved by the National Steering Committee
on
Sudden, Unexplained Infant Death

Endorsed by the
American Board of Medicolegal Death Investigators
National Association of Medical Examiners
National Sheriffs' Association

Project Manager
Terry W. Davis, EdD
Centers for Disease Control and Prevention

January 2007

Notes:

Table of Contents

Notes:

InfantDeathInvestigationGuidelines

Notes:

InvestigativeToolsandEquipment

1. Body bags or transport case (with ID tags).
2. Business cards/office cards with contact information.
3. Camera (digital).
4. Clean white linen sheet (stored in plastic bag).
5. Communication equipment (cell phone, pager, radio).
6. Disinfectant.
7. Evidence containers (paper bags, envelopes, containers, boxes, etc.).
8. Evidence tape and seal.
9. First aid kit.
10. Flashlight.
11. Gloves (universal precautions).
12. Hand lens (magnifying glass).
13. Investigative notebook.
14. Local maps.
15. Measurement instruments (tape measure, ruler, etc.).
16. Medical equipment kit (scissors, forceps, tweezers, swabs, etc.).
17. Official identification (for yourself).
18. Paper bags and envelopes.
19. Phone numbers (social services, child protection agencies, etc.).
20. Plastic trash bags.
21. Portable computer (laptop, pocket PC).
22. Portable lighting.
23. Reenactment doll.
24. Scene reporting forms (SUIDI Reporting Form or locally approved equivalent).
25. Specimen containers (for evidence items and toxicology specimens).
26. Tape and/or rubber bands.
27. Thermometer.
28. Voice recorder.
29. Watch.
30. Writing implements.

A

Notes:

Arriving at the Scene

1. Introduce and Identify Self and Role

Principle: Introductions at the scene allow the investigator to establish formal contact with all official agency representatives. Unlike most other death scenes, many infant deaths create multiple scenes, each requiring the investigator to communicate with people who have different roles and responsibilities. Emergency medical services (EMS), law enforcement, hospital, and daycare employees are all valuable investigative resources. The investigator must identify the first responder or agency contact to ascertain if any artifacts or contamination may have been introduced to, or removed from, the death scene. Investigators must work with other official personnel to ensure all scenes and key witnesses are identified before starting the investigation.

Procedure: Upon arrival at the scene, the investigator should

1. Identify the lead investigator at the scene and present identification.
2. Identify other essential officials at the scene (e.g., EMS, emergency department personnel, childcare providers, social/child protective services).
3. Explain the investigator's role in the investigation.
4. Identify and document the first essential official(s) to the scene (first "professional" arrival) for investigative follow-up.
5. Determine if the scene is safe to enter and conduct the investigation.

Summary: Infant death scenes can become crowded with emotional family members and witnesses. Introductions at the scene help establish a collaborative investigative effort with all professional participants. It is essential to carry official identification.

2. Exercise Scene Safety

Principle: Determining scene safety for all investigative personnel is essential to the investigative process. The risk of environmental and physical injury must be removed before starting a scene investigation. Environmental and chemical threats, hostile family members, and other witnesses may pose potential risks to investigators and must be controlled or removed from the scene before starting the investigation.

Procedure: Upon arrival at the scene, the investigator should

1. Secure the vehicle and park as safely as possible.
2. Assess or establish physical scene boundaries.
3. Identify incident command.
4. Use personal protective safety devices (as required).
5. Arrange for removal of animals or secure as necessary.
6. Obtain authorization to enter the scene from the person responsible for scene safety (e.g., law enforcement, fire marshal).
7. Observe and protect the integrity of the scene and evidence to the extent possible from contamination or loss by people, animals, and elements.

Note: Because of potential scene hazards (e.g., crowds, poisonous gases, traffic), the body may have to be removed before the scene investigation can continue.

Summary: Environmental and physical threats to the investigator must be removed in order to conduct a scene investigation safely. The investigator must endeavor to protect the evidence against contamination and loss.

3. Confirm or Pronounce Death

Principle: Appropriate personnel must make a determination of death before the death investigation is initiated. The confirmation or pronouncement of death determines jurisdictional responsibilities.

Procedure: Upon arrival at the scene, the investigator should

1. Locate and view the body.
2. Check for pulse, respiration, and reflexes, as appropriate.
3. Identify and document the person who made the official determination of death.
4. Document the time death was pronounced.
5. Ensure the death is pronounced, if required.

Summary: Once death has been determined, rescue/resuscitative efforts cease and medicolegal jurisdiction can be established. It is vital that this occur before the medical examiner/coroner assumes any responsibilities. If the infant was transported from the incident scene to the hospital, communicate with both EMS and emergency department personnel to determine where and when the death was "first" pronounced (i.e., infant dead at incident scene or transported to hospital, then pronounced).

4. Participate in Scene Briefing

Principle: The infant death investigation may involve multiple medical, legal, social, as well as public and private family health agency representatives. Scene investigators must recognize the varying jurisdictional and statutory responsibilities that apply to individual agency representatives and the role of each of the child-focused organizations involved with infant deaths. Determining each agency's role in the investigation and eventual follow-up is essential in planning the scope and depth of each scene investigation and the release of information to the public.

Procedure: Upon arrival at the scene, the investigator should

1. Locate the first responder and/or lead investigator.
2. Document the scene location consistent with other agencies.
3. Determine the nature and the scope of investigation by obtaining prelimi-nary investigative details (e.g., suspicious versus nonsuspicious death).
4. Identify and document witnesses and their relationship to the decedent.
5. Determine and document the individual(s) who last placed the infant down, last knew the infant was alive, and discovered the infant dead.
6. Ensure that initial accounts of the incident are obtained from the professional and nonprofessional responders.

Summary: EMS personnel are key resources at the scene briefing. Document their initial observations of witness reactions during the first minutes after their arrival. First responders' observations of unusual behavior, the removal of items from the scene, or people leaving the scene may prove valuable. The scene briefing allows for initial and factual information exchange between participating agency representatives. This includes scene location, time factors, initial witness information and behavior, agency responsibilities, investigative strategy, and follow-up activities.

5. Conduct Scene "Walk Through"

Principle: Conducting a scene "walk through" provides the investigator with an overview of the entire scene. The "walk through" allows the first opportunity to locate and view the environment where the infant was placed, last known alive, and found dead or unresponsive. In addition, items of evidentiary value may be identified, and initial investigative procedures can be established to ensure a systematic examination of the scene and body.

Procedure: To establish scene parameters and become familiar with the environment, the investigator should

1. Locate the first responder and/or lead investigator.
2. Determine the location where the infant was discovered dead or unresponsive.
3. Determine the location where the infant was last known alive.
4. Determine the location where the infant was placed.
5. Identify visible physical and fragile evidence.
6. Document and photograph fragile evidence immediately and collect, if appropriate.
7. Observe the physical living environment.
8. Locate and view the decedent, if possible.

Summary: Unlike most death investigations, the decedent in an infant death has almost always been moved since discovery. Therefore, it is essential that the investigator use this first opportunity to locate and evaluate the location(s) within the scene where the infant was purported to have been moved between placement and discovery, while also noting existing environmental conditions that may have affected the infant. The initial scene "walk through" is essential to minimize scene disturbance and prevent the loss or contamination of physical and fragile evidence.

6. Establish Chain of Custody

Principle: Ensuring the integrity of the evidence by establishing and maintaining a chain of custody is vital to an investigation. Documenting the collection and handling of all evidence and property will safeguard against subsequent allegations of tampering, theft, planting, and contamination of evidence.

Procedure: Throughout the investigation, those responsible for preserving the chain of custody should

1. Document the scene location and the investigator's time of arrival.
2. Determine the custodian(s) of evidence, the agency(ies) responsible for collecting specific types of evidence, and the evidence-collection priority for fragile/fleeting evidence.
3. Identify, secure, and preserve evidence with proper containers, labels, and preservatives.
4. Document the collection of evidence by recording its location at the scene, time of collection, and time and location of disposition.
5. Develop personnel lists, witness lists, and documentation of arrival and departure times for personnel.

Summary: It is essential to maintain a proper chain of custody for evidence. Through proper documentation, collection, and preservation, the integrity of the evidence can be assured. All items removed from the scene must be accounted for. Establishing and maintaining both evidence and property logs will reduce the likelihood of a challenge to the integrity of the evidence.

7. Follow Evidence-Collection Laws

Principle: The investigator must follow local, state, and federal laws for the collection of evidence to ensure its admissibility. The investigator must work collaboratively with all agency representatives to determine which agency has the legal authority to perform specific tasks related to collecting evidence.

Procedure: The investigator, before or upon arrival at the death scene, should work with other agencies to

1. Determine the need for a search warrant.
2. Determine each agency's legal investigative parameters.
3. Assign evidence-collection tasks based on legal parameters.
4. Document the collection of all evidence.
5. Document the collection of all items removed from the scene.

Summary: Following laws related to collecting evidence will ensure a complete and proper investigation in compliance with local, state, and federal laws, admissibility in court, and adherence to office policies and protocols. Witness statements obtained at the scene often prove to be the most significant pieces of evidence collected during the infant death investigation. These statements should be ascertained and documented by the professionals responsible and most qualified to do so.

Notes:

_____

_____

_____

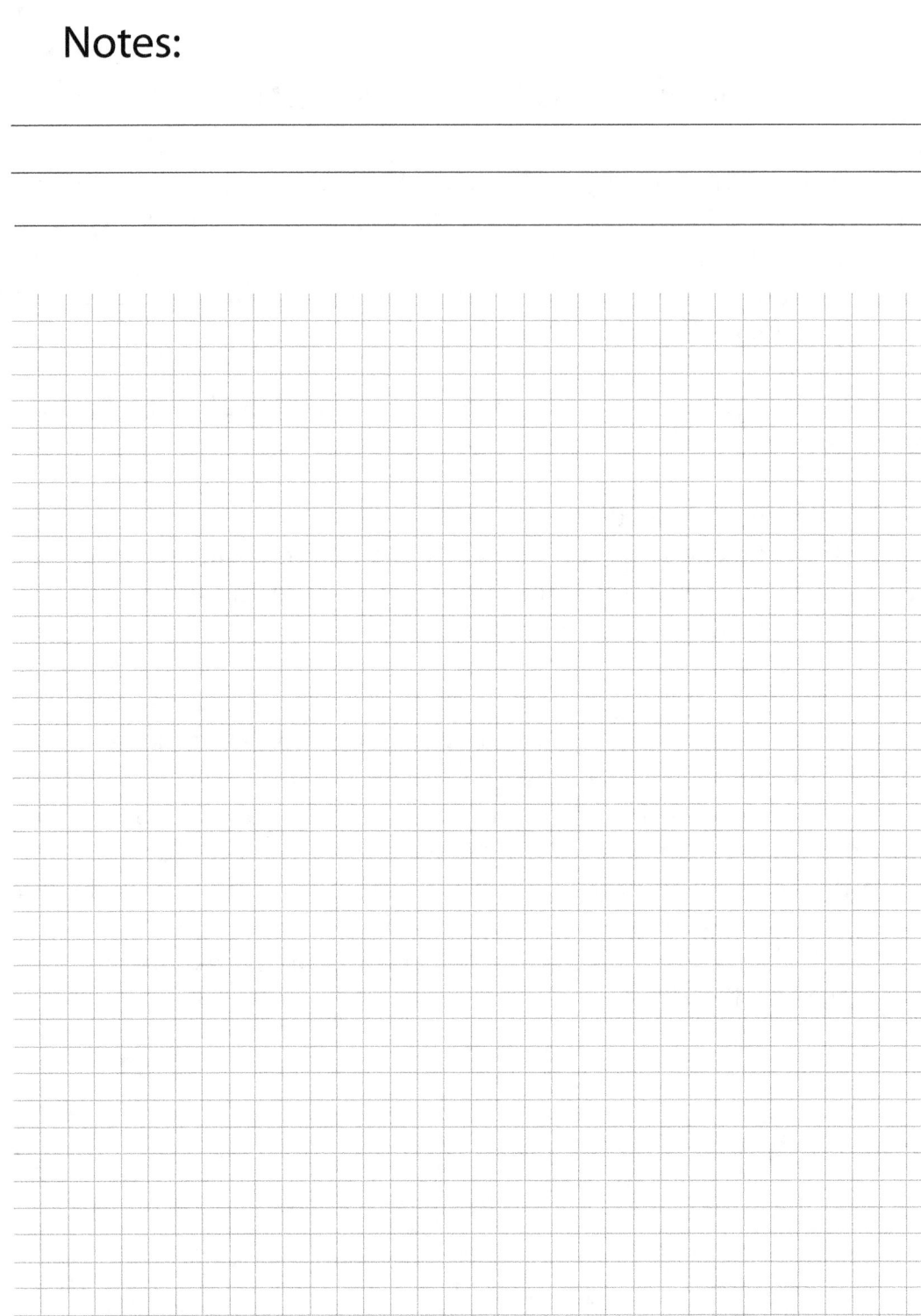

8. Photograph Scene

Principle: The photographic documentation of the scene creates a permanent historical record. If a forensic autopsy is performed, scene photographs are required to begin that procedure. Photographs taken at the scene provide forensic scientists with the details required to correlate scene findings with physical findings, and provide corroborating evidence that constructs a system of redundancy, should questions arise concerning the report, witness statements, or evidence.

Procedure: Before moving the body or evidence, or during the doll reenactment, the investigator should

1. Remove all nonessential personnel from the scene.
2. Obtain an overall (wide-angle) view of the scene to place the specific scene in its spatial context.
3. Photograph the immediate scene, showing environment.
4. Photograph a doll reenactment depicting placed and found positions, and locations within the scene environment.
5. Photograph all known and suspected sleeping surfaces.
6. Photograph items of environmental concern in relation to placed, last known alive, and found locations.
7. Obtain some photographs with scales.
8. Obtain photographs even if the body or other evidence has been removed or moved.

Note: Doll reenactment photographs assume movement of evidence and property. If the infant's body is present, document any movement.

Summary: Photography allows for the best permanent documentation of the death scene. It is essential that accurate scene photographs are available for the forensic pathologist, other investigators, agencies, and authorities to recreate the scene. It is essential that the investigator obtain accurate photographs before releasing the scene.

9. DevelopDescriptiveDocumentationofScene

Principle: Written documentation of the scene(s) provides a permanent record that may be used to correlate with and enhance photographic documentation, refresh recollections, and record observations.

Procedure: After photographic documentation of the scene and before evidence is removed, the investigator should

1. Document the residential environment, including the number of people living at the residence and its condition.
2. Diagram/describe in writing items of evidence and their relationship to the body in placed, last known alive, and found locations, with necessary measurements.
3. Describe and document, with measurements, blood and body-fluid evidence, including volume, patterns, spatters, and other characteristics.
4. Describe the scene environment, including odors, lights, temperatures, and other fragile evidence.
5. Describe powered appliances or devices present.
6. Write a descriptive caption for each photograph depicting a Sudden Unexplained Infant Death Investigation (SUIDI) Top 25 issue (see page 39) and provide to the pathologist before autopsy (if required).

Summary: Written documentation is essential to correlate with photographic evidence specific to the SUIDI Top 25 issues that typically affect infants and to provide that information to the pathologist before autopsy. Written documentation also assists police, other forensic scientists, and judicial and civil agencies with a legitimate interest in recreating the scene.

10. EstablishProbableLocationofInjuryorIllness

Principle: The location where the infant is first viewed by the investigator may not be the actual location where the injury/illness that contributed to the death occurred. It is imperative that the investigator attempt to determine the locations of any and all injury/illness that may have contributed to the death. Physical and environmental evidence at any and all locations (scenes) visited within 24 hours of death may be pertinent in establishing the cause, manner, and circumstances of an infant's death and should be considered "scenes."

Procedure: To obtain information regarding any and all probable locations associated with the infant's death, the investigator should

1. Identify the lead "professional" at the location where the body is first viewed.
2. Document the location where the death was confirmed.
3. Identify and record discrepancies in rigor mortis, livor mortis, and algor mortis.
4. Check the body, clothing, sleeping area, and overall scene for consistency/inconsistency of trace evidence and indicate artifact location(s).
5. Establish post-discovery activity (e.g., transport, interventions).
6. Document the location(s) of the infant within the prior 24 hours, and the method of transportation to and from each location.
7. Document the person(s) in contact with infant within the prior 24 hours, and their relationship to infant.
8. Conduct and document interviews with family members, EMS, law enforcement, health care providers, caregivers, and other witnesses.

Note: All interviews should be conducted by appropriate personnel, following proper legal procedures, and using appropriate interviewing techniques.

Summary: It is *uncommon* for the investigator to view the deceased infant in his or her "discovered" location and position. Family members, caregivers, EMS, medical and public safety personnel, and even witnesses have all been known to move and manipulate infants while attempting "resuscitation." This includes transporting the infant (alive or dead) from one location to another. In the interest of public health and safety, and to eliminate the possibility of criminal activity, each location must be investigated as a "scene" for evidence pertinent to cause and manner of death.

11. Collect, Inventory, and Safeguard Property a Evidence

Principle: Evidence related to the scene must be safeguarded by a chain of custody to ensure proper processing and availability for further evaluation. Property removed from the scene must be properly inventoried to ensure its eventual return to the parents or guardians.

Procedure: After property and evidence have been identified at the scene(s), the investigator (with a witness) should

1. Inventory, collect, and safeguard any illicit drugs or paraphernalia at the scene.
2. Inventory, collect, and safeguard any prescription medications at the scene and office.
3. Inventory, collect, and safeguard any nonprescription medications, including any home remedies at the scene and office.
4. Inventory, collect, and safeguard personal property or clothing at the scene and office.
5. Inventory, collect, and safeguard the infant's last known food source (e.g., bottles).
6. Inventory, collect, and safeguard any bedding, including sheets, pillows, and any other material the infant may have come into contact with.
7. Inventory, collect, and safeguard any portable devices that were in close proximity and in operation at the time of the infant's death.

Summary: Personal property and evidence are important items at any death scene. Evidence must be safeguarded to ensure its availability if needed for future evaluation and litigation. Personal property must be safeguarded to ensure its eventual return to the parents or guardians. Care must be taken to protect infant property, because the sentimental value to parents or guardians **cannot** be underestimated.

12. Interview Witness(es) at Scene

Principle: The documented statements of witnesses and their nonverbal behavior observed at the scene allows the investigator to obtain primary data regarding placement and discovery of the infant, as well as witness corroboration and history.

Procedure: Upon arrival at the scene, the investigator should

1. Identify and document statements from the first professional responders to the scene (e.g., EMS, law enforcement).
2. Obtain, confirm, and document the first professional responders' statements regarding the condition of the scene, body, and any treatments rendered.
3. Recover any written reports, notes, and lab samples (e.g., EMS run sheet, ED admission form) if available.
4. Collect all available identifying data on the witnesses (e.g., full name, address, DOB, work and home telephone numbers).
5. Establish the witnesses' relationship, residence, and association to the infant.
6. Identify the individual(s) who placed the infant, last knew infant was alive (LKA), and found the infant.
7. Obtain, confirm, and document all placement, LKA, and discovery histories regarding location, position, feeding.
8. Document any deviations from "normal" or "routine" infant behavior and activity within the last 24 hours.
9. Tape statements, if you have the appropriate equipment.

Summary: The final report must include the identity of witnesses and detailed statements from the individual(s) who placed, found, and can confirm the circumstances and time that the infant was last known to be alive. In addition, firsthand observations by responding agency representatives, and their written case documents, are essential in establishing the condition of the infant before the investigator's arrival at the scene. It is imperative that investigators be aware of any language barriers and cultural sensitivities that may exist. These interviews are delicate and must be conducted in a professional and sensitive manner, if any useful information is going to be obtained.

13.   Photograph Body and Doll Reenactment

Principle: The photographic documentation of the infant at the scene creates a permanent historical record of the body, the infant's terminal position, appearance, and any external trauma. When the infant's body has been moved, doll reenactments allow for the visualization and documentation of the infant's initial placed position, and discovered position.

Procedure: Upon arrival at the scene, the investigator should

1.   Photograph the infant as found and the immediate scene.
2.   Using a doll reenactment, document the position in which the infant was placed and found (with placer and finder, if possible).
3.   Photograph the sleeping surface beneath the body for any evidence of secretions, surface indentations, or pockets.
4.   In the case of photographs taken at the hospital, attempt to document the presence of trauma, if any, resuscitative treatments, and general external appearance of the body (e.g., livor, rigor, petechiae).
5.   Take additional photographs after removing items that interfere with photographic documentation of the infant (e.g., bedding, toys).
6.   Create a body diagram indicating the approximate location of all markings and trauma on the body.
7.   Report SUIDI Top 25 documentation to the pathologist.

Summary: Photographing the body documents its position and appearance. However, finding an infant in its actual found position at the scene is uncommon, since caregivers understandably initiate resuscitative measures and disrupt the scene. In addition, emergency response personnel further disrupt the scene when attempting resuscitation, frequently removing the infant from the scene, making photography of the actual found position impossible. Regardless, the investigator can, with the assistance of witnesses, document body position using the doll reenactment and report critical pre-autopsy data to the pathologist.

14. Conduct the External Body Examination (superficial)

Principle: Conducting the external examination documents the infant's physical characteristics, relationship to the scene, and injuries, if present. This documentation (photographic and graphic [on body diagram form]) provides detailed information about the possible cause, manner, and circumstances of death.

Procedure: Upon arrival at the scene, the investigator should

1. Document the infant's physical characteristics (e.g., height, state of hydration, cleanliness).
2. Document the presence, condition, and cleanliness of clothing.
3. Document the presence of body rashes.
4. Document the presence of marks or scars.
5. Document the presence or absence of injury/trauma (e.g., grab marks, bite marks, burns).
6. Document treatment or resuscitative efforts.
7. Determine the need for further evaluation/assistance of forensic specialists.

Summary: External examination of the infant provides information about the state of care, injuries, and presence of illness. Although injuries may not be visible on the external surface of the body, their presence immediately alerts the investigator to the possibility of an unnatural death. All findings specific to SUIDI Top 25 issues should be reported to the pathologist before autopsy. In addition, the external examination may alert the investigator to abnormal states of infant growth and development.

15. Preserve Evidence (On Body)

Principle: Generating photographic and written documentation of evidence on the body allows the investigator to create a permanent historical record of that evidence. To maintain chain of custody, evidence must be collected, preserved, and transported properly. In addition to any physical evidence visible on the body and bedding, blood and other body fluids present must be photographed and documented before collection and transport. Fragile evidence (that which can be easily contaminated, lost, or altered) must also be documented.

Procedure: Upon arrival at the scene, the investigator should

1. Photograph and document evidence of trauma (e.g., bite marks).
2. Photograph and document the body's physical condition (e.g., diaper rash) and cleanliness.
3. Photograph and document the clothing, its condition, and its cleanliness.
4. Photograph and document evidence of resuscitative efforts and equipment.
5. Collect trace evidence before transporting the body.
6. Arrange for the collection and transport of evidence at the scene.
7. Ensure the proper collection of blood and body fluids for subsequent analysis (if body will be released from the scene to an outside agency without autopsy).

Summary: It is essential that evidence be identified, collected, preserved, transported, and documented in an orderly and proper fashion to ensure reliable analysis and a defensible chain of custody, should admissibility in a legal action occur. The preservation and documentation of the evidence must be initiated by the investigator at the scene to prevent alterations or contamination. Photographs of evidence on the body that depict a SUIDI Top 25 issue must be reported to the pathologist *before* autopsy.

16. Establish Infant Identification

Principle: Establishing or confirming the identification of an infant and his or her parents or guardians is paramount to the death investigation. Proper identification allows notification of the next of kin, aids in the investigation, and allows the death certificate to be completed properly.

Procedure: To establish identity, the investigator should document use of the following methods:

1. Direct visual or photographic identification of the infant, if visually recognizable.
2. Comparison of clothing, personal effects, or evidence at the scene.
3. Scientific methods such as DNA comparisons.
4. Circumstantial methods such as personal effects, circumstances, physical features, and any unique characteristics.
5. Search of national, state, and local missing children's databases (e.g., National Center for Missing and Exploited Children).

Summary: Infant identification when the next of kin are present at the death scene is straightforward and uncomplicated. However, if an infant is discovered by strangers or is unclaimed, identification can be problematic, because fingerprints and dental comparisons are not available options. In these cases, the investigator must document all descriptive features, physical description, and any unique anomalies or evidence.

17. Document Postmortem Changes

Principle: Documenting postmortem changes to the body, when correlated with circumstantial information, can assist investigators in estimating the approximate time of death. Inconsistencies between postmortem changes and body location may indicate movement of the body and validate or invalidate witness statements. This information is essential to the pathologist *before* the autopsy begins.

Procedure: Upon arrival at the scene, the investigator should observe, photograph, and graphically document (i.e., on body diagram form)

1. Livor (color, location, blanchability, Tardieu spots) consistent/inconsistent with position of body.
2. Rigor (stage/intensity, location on the body, broken, inconsistent with the scene).
3. Degree of decomposition (putrefaction, adipocere, mummification, skeletonization, as appropriate).
4. Insect and animal activity.
5. Scene temperature: inside and outside (document method used and time estimated).
6. Description of body temperature (e.g., warm, cold, frozen) or measurement of body temperature (document method used and time of measurement).

Summary: The onset of postmortem changes can occur more rapidly in infants than in adults; therefore, documenting the time that the observations were made is essential. Investigators need to solicit information from the first responding agency representatives (e.g., EMS, law enforcement) or hospital emergency department personnel, to collect and document vital sign information and the appearance of the infant when first viewed.

18. Participate in Scene Debriefing

Principle: The scene debriefing helps investigators from all participating agencies to establish post-scene responsibilities by sharing data regarding particular scene findings. The scene debriefing provides each agency the opportunity for input, special requests for assistance, additional information, special examinations, and other requests requiring interagency communication, cooperation, and education.

Procedure: Before leaving the scene, the investigator should meet with other official agency representatives to

1. Confirm the birth mother's date of birth.
2. Contact local child protective services to determine any previous reports of abuse or neglect.
3. Evaluate the potential safety of other children at the residence (in suspected abuse cases).
4. Determine whether a specialist (e.g., pediatric radiologist) is needed to assist in the investigation.
5. Share critical investigative data (pre-autopsy reporting to the pathologist – SUIDI Top 25).
6. Review caregiver background(s) (e.g., babysitter, licensing of daycare, foster care).
7. Contact public health agency (if communicable disease is suspected).
8. Communicate special requests to other appropriate agencies, being mindful of the necessity for confidentiality.

Summary: The scene debriefing is the best opportunity for investigative participants to communicate special requests and to confirm all current and additional scene data and responsibilities. The debriefing allows for the confirmation of infant details and parental information, coordination of post-scene activities, and scheduling of follow-up activities, if necessary.

19. Determine Notification Procedures (Next of Kin)

Principle: Parents or guardians are not always present at the scene of an infant death. Every reasonable effort should be made to notify them as soon as possible. Investigators may enlist the support of a local bereavement agency, using a "team" approach for the actual notification. The notification initiates the closure process for the family, helps determine disposition of remains, and facilitates the collection of additional information relative to the case.

Procedure: If the parents/guardians are absent from the scene, the investigator should

1. Identify the parents/guardians (determine who will perform this task if identity is not readily apparent).
2. Locate the parents/guardians (determine who will perform this task).
3. Contact the local infant death support agency for possible assistance with the notification.
4. Notify the parents/guardians (assign individuals to perform this task) and record time of notification, or, if delegated to another agency, gain confirmation when notification is made.
5. Notify concerned agencies of the status of the notification.
6. Document the notification in the case file.

Summary: If the parents or guardians are not at the scene, the investigator is responsible for ensuring that they are identified, located, and notified as quickly as possible. Making an infant death notification corroboratively with a local support agency professional is often advisable. The time and method of notification should be documented. Failure to locate the parents/guardians and efforts to do so should be a matter of record. This ensures that a diligent effort has been made to contact the family.

20. Ensure Security of Remains

Principle: Ensuring the security of the body requires the investigator to perform or supervise the removal of the infant from the scene in a sensitive and caring manner. Appropriate chain of custody is maintained to preclude misidentification upon receipt at the examining agency. This function also includes safeguarding all potential physical evidence and/or property and clothing that remain on the body.

Procedure: Before leaving the scene, the investigator should

1. Ensure that the body is protected from further trauma or contamination (if not, document) and unauthorized removal of therapeutic and resuscitative equipment.
2. Inventory and secure property, clothing, and personal effects that are on the body (remove in a controlled environment with a witness present).
3. Identify property and clothing to be retained as evidence (in a controlled environment).
4. Carefully wrap the infant (as if alive) in a clean sheet or blanket.
5. Carry the infant's body (as if alive) from the scene to the transport vehicle.
6. Carefully place and secure the infant's body in the passenger compartment of the vehicle and use the infant body bag/transport case as necessary during transit.

NOTE: The infant's body must be removed from the scene in a caring and respectful manner. Parents, caregivers, and/or witnesses will note the behavior and actions of the investigator while this task is performed.

Summary: Ensuring the security of the remains facilitates proper identification of the remains, maintains a proper chain of custody, and safeguards property and evidence. The infant must be handled and transported from the scene as if it were alive. To avoid damaging tissues and creating artifacts, the recovery of blood and other body fluids should be deferred to the pathologist at the autopsy.

21. Document Discovery History

Principle: The investigation of an infant death begins with the circumstances of the discovery history. This basic information will dictate the direction of the subsequent investigation, jurisdiction, and authority. The focus (breadth/depth) of further investigation depends on this information.

Procedure: To correctly document and report the discovery history, the investigator should:

1. Identify and record the person(s) who found the infant dead or unresponsive.
2. Document the circumstances surrounding the discovery (use doll reenactment).
3. Verify markings and trauma placed on the body diagram.
4. Report discovery history to pathologist (pre-autopsy report).

Summary: Information in the discovery history that is inconsistent with information gathered in the subsequent investigation (e.g., from autopsy, child protective services, EMS observations) may be of paramount importance to determining cause and manner of death. The investigator must ensure that all data are collected systematically and reported to the pathologist before the autopsy.

E

22. Document Terminal Episode History

Principle: The circumstances and events that surround the infant's death play a significant role in determining cause and manner of death. Documenting medical interventions or procuring antemortem specimens from emergency medical personnel help establish the infant's medical condition or activities before death.

Procedure: To determine the sequence of events occurring before the infant's death, the investigator should

1. Document the circumstances surrounding the placement of the infant (using a doll reenactment).
2. Document when, where, how, and by whom the infant was last known alive (LKA).
3. Document any incidents or injuries within 24 hours preceding death.
4. Document any complaints, symptoms, or illnesses within 24 hours preceding death.
5. Document infant exposure to sick people within 24 hours preceding death.
6. Review and obtain a copy of EMS records and actions.
7. Obtain copies of relevant medical records.
8. Obtain antemortem specimens (if available).

Summary: Obtaining the infant's medical history and records of the circumstances preceding the infant's death distinguishes medical treatment from trauma. This history and relevant antemortem specimens assist the medical examiner/coroner in determining cause and manner of death.

23. Document Infant Medical History

Principle: An infant's medical records and history frequently contain information important to the investigation. The medical information assists in identifying elements that may have caused the death. Signs and symptoms of medical illness as well as previous exposures to illnesses may assist the pathologist in determining the cause of death.

Procedure: Through interviews and review of written records, the investigator should

1. Document prenatal history (e.g., doctor visits, mother's health).
2. Document birth history (e.g., infant gestational age, birth complications).
3. Document healthcare provider information (e.g., name, institution, contact number).
4. Document infant exposure to maternal drug and alcohol abuse.
5. Obtain information regarding any symptoms of medical illness or exposure within 24 hours preceding death.
6. Document administration of any drugs or home remedies.
7. Contact the treating physician or hospitals to confirm medical history and treatments (e.g., immunizations, illnesses, growth).

Summary: Obtaining a thorough infant medical history, including prenatal, delivery, and postnatal information, allows the investigator to focus the investigation and alert the pathologist to possible congenital birth anomalies, inherited errors of metabolism, and other complications or illnesses that may have contributed to the death or require additional study and investigation.

24. DocumentCaregiverMentalHealthHistory

Principle: The mental health of the caregiver may be a factor in the infant's death. Gaining insight into the caregiver's state of mind and ability to care for an infant may produce clues that will aid in establishing the cause, manner, and circumstances of the death.

Procedure: The investigator shall obtain information from sources familiar with the caregiver's mental health history to

1. Document the caregiver's state of mind at the time of the death (e.g., agitated, depressed, frustrated, exhausted).
2. Document the reaction of the caregiver to the infant's death.
3. Determine the infant's temperament, behavior, and daily care requirements.
4. Determine the caregiver's previous diagnoses of depression or other mental illness from family, friends, and acquaintances.
5. Assess the caregiver's potential mental health stressors (e.g., single parent, lack of education, young age, lack of family support system, financial instability).
6. "Rate" the caregiver's perceived level of stress related to caring for the infant.
7. Ascertain the extent of the caregiver's use of drugs and alcohol.
8. Determine whether the caregiver requires access to mental health services and refer if indicated.

Summary: Assessing the mental health of the caregiver allows the investigator to determine the role that these factors may have played in the infant's death. Because of the stressful nature of an infant death, investigators arriving at the scene need to assess the mental state of the caregiver and provide access to services if warranted.

25. Document Caregiver Social History

Principle: The social history of the caregiver includes marital, family, educational, employment, and financial information of the infant's primary caregiver(s). The caregiver's daily routines, habits, activities, friends, and associates help develop a caregiver profile. This information may assist the investigator in establishing cause, manner, and circumstances of an infant's death.

Procedure: When collecting relevant social history, the investigator should

1. Identify the primary caregiver(s).
2. Document the marital/domestic history of primary caregiver(s).
3. Document the employment history.
4. Document the daily routines, habits, and activities, including those of any additional caregiver(s) of the infant.
5. Document the caregiver's friends, associates, and relatives who may be associated with the infant.
6. Document religious and ethnic affiliations or practices. Assess any religious objections to the autopsy.
7. Document caregiver's level of education.
8. Determine the residence length and previous residences.
9. Document any criminal history or previous contacts to child protection agencies.

Summary: Assessing the social history of the caregiver gives the investigator a view of the infant's immediate environment and potential for exposure to harmful people, places, and things.

Notes:

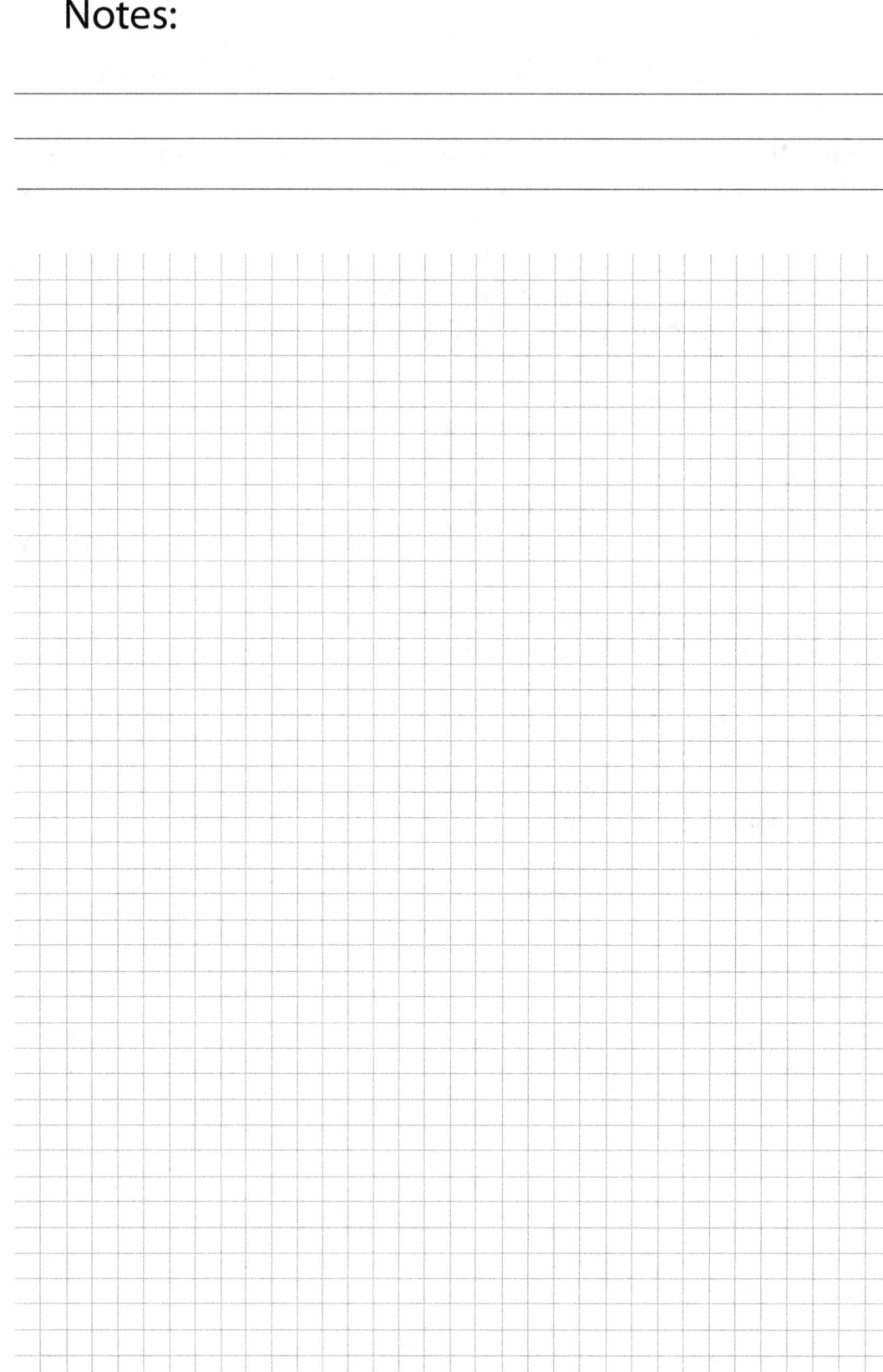

26. Maintain Jurisdiction Over Body

Principle: Maintaining jurisdiction of the infant's body allows the investigator to protect the chain of custody as the infant is transported from the scene for autopsy, specimen collection, or storage.

Procedure: When maintaining jurisdiction over the body, the investigator should

1. Arrange for and document secure transportation of the body to a medical or autopsy facility for further examination or storage.
2. Coordinate and document procedures to be performed when the body is received at the facility (e.g., radiology, serology testing).
3. Provide the family with written documentation of procedures, along with contact names and numbers.
4. Transport the body in a sensitive and caring fashion.

Summary: By providing secure transportation of the body from the scene to an authorized receiving facility, the investigator maintains jurisdiction and protects chain of custody of the body.

F

27. Release Jurisdiction of Body

Principle: The investigator releases jurisdiction of the body after examination by the pathologist. Before releasing jurisdiction of the infant to the family or funeral director, to the investigator should contact the person responsible for certifying the death to review the circumstances of the death. The investigator verifies all information required to complete the death certificate, including demographic information, date, time, and location of death.

Procedure: When releasing jurisdiction over the body, the investigator should

1. Determine who will sign the death certificate (name, title, agency, contact information, etc.).
2. Review case circumstances with the certifier to support release of the body (i.e., do they agree with the investigator's assessment of the case?).
3. Collect and secure any evidence before the body is released from the scene.
4. Document and arrange with the funeral director to reconcile all death certificate information.
5. Release the body to a funeral director or other authorized receiving agent.
6. Inform the parent/guardian of the infant's transfer to the funeral director.

Summary: The investigator releases jurisdiction of the infant only after determining who will sign the death certificate; documenting the date, time, and location of death; collecting appropriate specimens; and releasing the body to the funeral director or other authorized receiving agent. It is also good practice to provide the certifier with an overview of the case to ensure that releasing the body is supported.

28. Perform Exit Procedures

Principle: Bringing formal closure to the scene investigation ensures that important evidence has been collected and the scene has been processed. A systematic review of the scene ensures that artifacts or equipment are not inadvertently left behind, dangerous materials or conditions have been reported, and that the family or caregiver has a support network available before they are left alone.

Procedure: When performing exit procedures, the investigator should

1. Identify, inventory, and remove all evidence collected at the scene.
2. Remove all personal equipment and material from the scene.
3. Report and document any dangerous material or conditions.
4. Remind family members or caregivers of any follow-up activities they may be involved in.
5. Inform agency representatives (e.g., EMS, law enforcement, hospital) of any follow-up activities they may be involved in.
6. Contact child protection authorities immediately if other children are present and abuse is suspected.
7. Inform the parents/guardians of your destination and route (if necessary).
8. Ensure that the parents/guardians have the emotional support necessary to be left alone.

Summary: Conducting a scene "walk through" upon exit ensures that all evidence has been collected, materials are not inadvertently left behind, any dangerous materials or conditions have been reported to the proper entities, and the family is supported.

29. Assist Family

Principle: The investigator provides the family with a timetable so they can arrange for final disposition of the infant, and information on available community resources that may assist the family.

Procedure: Before leaving the scene, the investigator should

1. Inform the family if an autopsy may be required or that an evaluation will be conducted.
2. Inform the family of available support services (e.g., infant bereavement agencies, critical incident stress) for assistance and questions.
3. Ensure that the family has an adequate support network before leaving them alone.
4. Provide the family with an approximate investigative timetable (e.g., release of autopsy or toxicology results).
5. Inform the family of the approximate time for release of the body.
6. Inform the family of available reports, including costs, if any.
7. Provide the family with contact numbers for local support groups/agencies.

Summary: The interaction with the family allows the investigator to assist and direct them to appropriate resources. It is essential that families be given a timetable of events so that they can begin making any necessary arrangements. In addition, the investigator needs to make them aware of what information will be available to them and when that information will be available to be picked up.

Notes:

Notes:

Notes:

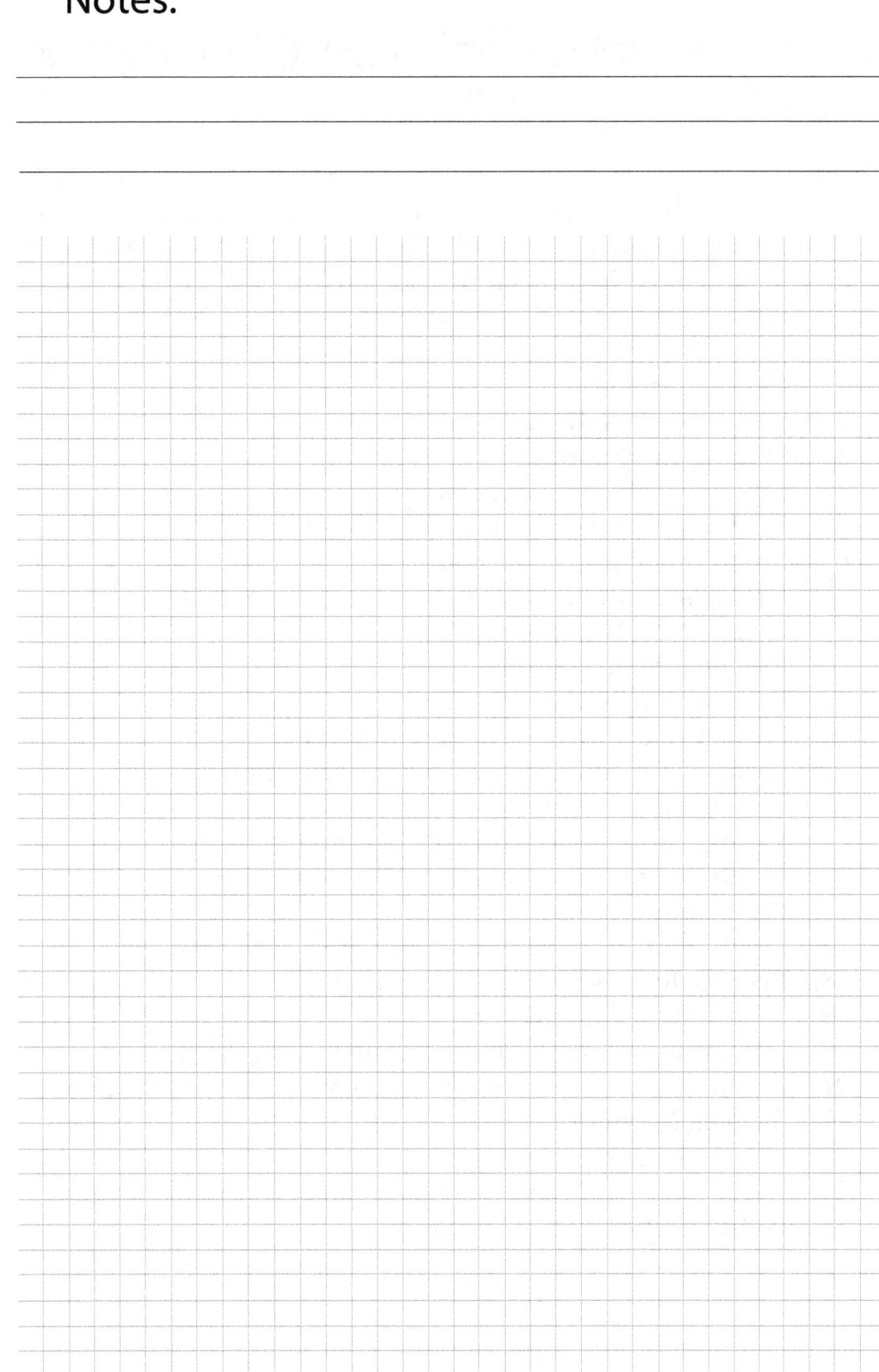

Sudden,UnexplainedInfantDeathInvestigation
SUIDI Top 25

Forensic pathologists consider the following information critical to determining the cause and manner of death in the investigation of sudden, unexplained infant death. The following scene/case information should be collected and provided to the forensic pathologist BEFORE the forensic autopsy is performed.

1. Case information
2. Evidence of asphyxia
3. Sharing sleep surfaces
4. Change in sleep conditions
5. Evidence of hyperthermia/hypothermia
6. Environmental scene hazards
7. Unsafe sleeping conditions
8. Diet or recent change in diet
9. Recent hospitalizations
10. Previous medical diagnosis
11. History of acute life-threatening events
12. History of medical care — without diagnosis
13. Recent fall or other injury
14. History of religious, cultural, or ethnic remedies
15. Death due to natural causes other than SIDS
16. Prior sibling deaths
17. Previous encounters with police or social service agencies
18. Request for tissue or organ donation
19. Objection to autopsy
20. Pre-terminal resuscitative treatment
21. Death due to trauma (injury), poisoning, or intoxication
22. Suspicious circumstances
23. Other alerts for pathologist's attention
24. Description of the circumstances surrounding the death
25. Pathologist contact information

InfantDeathInvestigationGuidelines

Investigative Tools
and Equipment

Arriving at the Scene

Documenting and
Evaluating the Scene

Documenting and
Evaluating the Body

Establishing Infant
Profile Information

Completing the
Scene Investigation